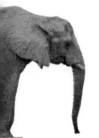

Mnemonics
for Paediatrics

Munib Haroon BSc MBChB MRCPCH MMedSci
Specialist Registrar in Paediatrics
Yorkshire Deanery

PasTest
Dedicated to your success

© 2006 PASTEST LTD
Egerton Court
Parkgate Estate
Knutsford
Cheshire
WA16 8DX

Telephone: 01565 752000

First Published 2006

ISBN: 1 904627 90 0
ISBN: 978 1 904627 906

A catalogue record for this book is available from the British Library.

The information contained within this book was obtained by the author from
reliable sources. However, while every effort has been made to ensure its
accuracy, no responsibility for loss, damage or injury occasioned to any person
acting or refraining from action as a result of information contained herein can be
accepted by the publishers or author.

PasTest Revision Books and Intensive Courses

PasTest has been established in the field of postgraduate medical education
since 1972, providing revision books and intensive study courses for doctors
preparing for their professional examinations.

Books and courses are available for the following specialties:

**MRCGP, MRCP Parts 1 and 2, MRCPCH Parts 1 and 2, MRCPsych,
MRCS, MRCOG Parts 1 and 2, DRCOG, DCH, FRCA, PLAB Parts 1 and 2.**

For further details contact:

PasTest, Freepost, Knutsford, Cheshire WA16 7BR

Tel: 01565 752000   **Fax: 01565 650264**
www.pastest.co.uk   **enquiries@pastest.co.uk**

Text typeset and designed by Type Study, Scarborough, North Yorkshire

Printed and bound in the UK by MPG Books Ltd, Bodmin, Cornwall

Mnemonic

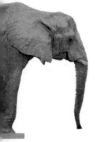

1753, from the Greek *mnemonikos* 'of or pertaining to memory,' from *mnemon* (gen. *mnemonos*) 'remembering, mindful,' from *mnasthai* 'remember.'

Mnemosyne, lit. 'memory, remembrance,' was a Titaness, mother of the Muses.

Contents

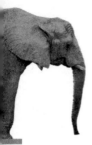

About the author

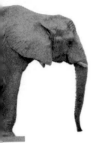

Munib Haroon BSc MBChB MRCPCH MMedSci
Munib trained at Leeds University and has subsequently trained
in paediatrics throughout the Yorkshire region. He is interested in
academic paediatrics and medical education and is currently a
Specialist Registrar at the Yorkshire Deanery.

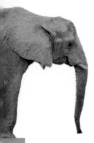

Acknowledgments

The conception and the gestational stage of this book proceeded without complications thanks to the suggestions and advice of Sophie Haroon.

I am grateful to Amy Smith, Kirsten Baxter and the staff at PasTest who ensured the safe delivery of this book at term.

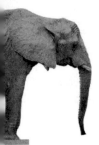

Introduction

Mnemonics and their making

Which nerve roots innervate the diaphragm?

When over 20 doctors who had been out of medical school for several years were recently asked this question they ALL remembered that the nerve roots in question were C3,4,5. Not only that, but the reason they stated for being able to remember this fact was that they had all learnt a mnemonic at medical school, '3,4,5 keeps the diaphragm alive'. A good point at which to start when trying to illustrate the usefulness of mnemonics.

Though in some quarters mnemonics are waved away dismissively as being 'a cheat' or in more medical education circles as 'facilitating a surface approach to learning rather than a deep one' they have a great heritage going back to ancient times.

The etymology of the word is a Greek word which means 'pertaining to the memory' while Mnemosyne was the Greek goddess of memory and the mother of the Muses.

So there you have it, a learning technique with great classical roots which also happens to be effective.

In medicine, mnemonics have long been popular especially in subjects such as anatomy and subjects which seem to be based on memorising lots of information in a short space of time for effective regurgitation at the 2nd MBs.

Paediatrics is a broad subject which students encounter at medical school and later on in post-graduate training. It has seemed to me that the technique of mnemonics has been under utilised by paediatricians and would be of use to those learning the subject at whatever level, be it at medical school or as an SHO revising for post-graduate exams. A mnemonic is essentially a 'tool' or device which helps with the retention of information.

The device for remembering the innervation of the diaphragm as illustrated above is one such mnemonic which incorporates the information into a brief and memorable rhyme.

Being a person who has an interest in mnemonics I have classified them up into 4 varieties, and for ease of memorisation have called them types 1, 2, 3 and 4.

Type 1

This is the acronym, and one of the commonest types of mnemonic. For example, if a baby goes blue on the ventilator, neonatologists remember the word DOPE. This acronym consists of four letters, each of which stands for a cause which may be causing the baby to go blue.

Thus; **D** **D**isplacement of the tube
O **O**bstruction
P **P**neumothorax
E **E**quipment failure.

This is quite easy to remember and highly useful at 4 am when dragged half asleep onto a neonatal intensive care unit, and also when confronted with the situation in the more artificial circumstances of an exam paper.

Now obviously these aren't the ONLY causes but they are the main causes. The idea with mnemonics as we shall reiterate is to keep them simple.

Other variations of this theme are seen. Some mnemonics don't actually spell out a word, but instead make use of some other combination of letters which are easy to remember, or make use of sequences of memorable numbers.

Such as the vowels, **AEIOU**.

Each letter has been used to represent one of the causes of coma.

Apoplexy, **E**pilepsy, **I**nfection, **O**xygen, **U**rea.

As you can see writing mnemonics takes a bit of imagination, and remembering them requires you to understand that use is made of 'proxies', in other words a word like urea represents generic 'metabolic conditions' rather than urea itself being a cause of coma. This above mnemonic also demonstrates to us that a lot of mnemonics use a broad brush when thinking of differentials. The use of mnemonics is to give you a hook to 'hang your coat' or differentials on, not to help you remember all 35 causes of a coma.

Type 2

The sentence

Never **E**at **S**hredded **W**heat – the four points of a compass and their order, ie **N**orth **E**ast **S**outh **W**est.

Okay so there you have it, the one we all learnt as a schoolchild, and if you are not familiar with that one then maybe you remember the medical one about 'ten zombies b*gger*ng your cat?' A picturesque though unfeline way to remember the branches of the facial nerve. Here each word, or rather the first letter (or so) stands for another surrogate word. Never for North, eat for East, etc etc.

Type 3

The poem

'Thirty days hath September'

This requires a bit more imagination to construct and needs to be extremely memorable and easy to remember, and hence is not seen that often; when done well however it can't be beaten as an aid and sticks in the mind for many years.

Type 4

Type 4 is the hybrid of the above types.

Its usefulness arises because it is all very well constructing a mnemonic such as DOPE for the causes of the blue ventilated baby, except that it does leave you with the problem of how you are going to associate the word DOPE with the concept of the blue baby. In other words how will you remember what the mnemonic DOPE is for. Is it for the causes of renal failure or the causes of cough?

The way this is overcome is by knitting one mnemonic inside another.

Thus:

'A baby blue has got no hope
If you forget to think of DOPE.'

Okay, now we know that DOPE is associated with the baby who goes blue on the ventilator. Thus this combination of types 1 and 4 should be easier to remember than the word DOPE on its own.

How to write mnemonics.

The above discussion has been done to enable you to think about mnemonics when you encounter them and also to help you devise your own.

I know what you are thinking, surely this is a book of mnemonics and not *about* mnemonics? And if so why is he telling us to write our own?

Well a lot of people have thought long and hard about mnemonics over the years and have come to the conclusion that the best mnemonics are usually those which are:

1. Rude
2. Funny
3. Basic
4. Relevant to you
5. Self written
6. All of the above.

Over the years I have written a lot of mnemonics, a few of these I have deliberately not incorporated because they will mean very little to you (for instance a mnemonic based on my date of birth will mean nothing to you unless you happen to be a person who is going to send me a birthday card). Similarly the most memorable mnemonics that I have come across in anatomy are some of the most rudest (and funniest) and alas many a publisher would be reluctant to print them. Nevertheless do not go away from the introduction thinking 'this book should be called DIY mnemonics' as I promise that I will list hundreds of them, all of which I think are very effective, because they are funny, basic or rude but within the acceptable boundaries of publish-ability. But the point that needs to be made is that often the most effective mnemonics are those you devise yourself.

The book is divided into chapters based on systems.

I have first listed the mnemonic and the information to which it pertains and added brief notes so the book can stand on its own as a revision book. As I have mentioned earlier, the mnemonics are aids to learning – they are *not* comprehensive.

I have found mnemonics useful ever since I went to medical school and still use them; I thus hope that medical students as well as doctors will find this book useful.

Munib Haroon

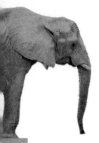

Abbreviations

ASD	Atrial septal defect
CF	Cystic fibrosis
ECMO	Extracorporeal membrane oxygenation
ET	Endotracheal tube
GI	Gastrointestinal
GU	Genitourinary
MAS	Meconium aspiration syndrome
NSAIDS	Non-steroidal anti-inflammatory drugs
PDA	Patent ductus arteriosus
PPHN	Persistent pulmonary hypertension of the newborn
RDS	Respiratory distress syndrome
RTA	Renal tubular acidosis
TAPVD	Total anomalous pulmonary venous drainage
TTN	Transient tachypnoea of the newborn
TB	Tuberculosis
VSD	Ventricular septal defect

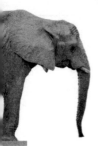

1. Respiratory paediatrics

1.1 Embryology

A. The embryological development of the lungs occurs in five stages:

Embryonic	**Even**	**Emma**
↓	↓	↓
PSeudoglandular	**psychotic**	**says**
↓	↓	↓
Canalicular	**canaries**	**can I lick a**
↓	↓	↓
Saccular	**suck seeds**	**sac**
↓	↓	↓
Alveolar	**a lot**	**Albert?**

So you can remember either 'Even psychotic canaries suck seeds a lot' or 'Emma says can I lick a sac Albert?'

The length of each stage in weeks (approximately) can be remembered by the sequence 5, 10, 10, 10, 5.

5, 10, 10, 10, 5

And if you add them all up it equals 40, ie the 40 weeks of gestation.

1.2 Symptoms and signs of respiratory disease

A. Assessment of the child with respiratory distress

When assessing the child with respiratory distress, you **assess the whEEEze**

Effort
Efficacy
Effect

---

notes

Effort

Recession
Respiratory rate
Grunting
Use of accessory muscles
Nasal flaring

Efficacy

Breath sounds
Chest expansion/ abdominal excursion

Effects of inadequate breathing

Heart rate
Skin colour
Mental status
Oxygen saturation

B. The signs of life threatening asthma are:

Asthmatics die on the seven seas (c's)

Cyanosis
Confusion
Collapse/**C**onked out. (ie exhaustion)
Cilent **C**hest
CO$_2$ climbs (but may be normal)

C. Clubbing

Clubbing makes you look CRAP

Cardiac
Respiratory
Abdominal
Paternal (ie familial)

D. Respiratory clubbing

ABCDEF

A	Abscess
B	Bronchiectasis
C/d	Cystic (fibrosis) disease
E	Empyema
F	Fibrosing alveolitis

E. Chronic cough

When there's a cough in the nursery, rock the babes IN CRADLEs

IN	Infections
C	Cystic fibrosis
R	Rings, slings and airway things
A	Aspiration
D	Dyskinetic cilia
L	Lung/airway/vascular malformations
E	oEsophageal reflux

F. Wheeze

There's no VACCINE for a wheeze

V	Virus
A	Asthma
C	Cardiac
C	Cystic
IN	INfection
E	AllErgy/oEdema

1.3 Causes and conditions

A. Neonatal respiratory distress

S.O.B. NACHARS (knackers) neonates

N pNeumonia
A Aspiration
C Cardiac/Congenital
H (pulmonary) Hypertension
A Airway problem
R RDS
S Surgical lesion

B. The neonate who goes blue on the ventilator

A baby blue has got no hope

If you don't even think of DOPE!

D Displacement
O Obstruction
P Pneumothorax
E Equipment failure

C. Causes of a pleural effusion

3 Hs, 3 Cs, 3 Is

H Heart failure, Hypoproteinaemic states, Hypothyroidism
C Constrictive pericarditis, Connective tissue disease, Consumption (TB)
I Infection, Infarction, Intestinal (ie inflammation from abdomen, ie pancreatitis)

NB The Hs are the causes where the effusion has a low protein content (<30 g/l). We remember this as the **H** contains the **h**ypoproteinaemic state. Constrictive pericarditis is also a cause of a hypoproteinaemic effusion.

notes

> Effusions are divided into exudates and transudates.
>
> Can be distinguished by protein content.
>
> Transudate protein content <30gm/L
>
> Exudate protein content >30gm/L
>
> The H's are the causes where the effusion has a low protein content (<30gm/l) we remember this as the H contains the hypoproteinaemic state.
>
> Constrictive pericarditis is also a cause of a hypoproteinaemic effusion.

D. Causes of a false-positive sweat test

The Sweaty CAGED MAID is positively false!!!

C A	**C**ongenital **A**drenal hyperplasia
G	**G**lycogen storage diseases
E D	**E**ctodermal **D**ysplasia/eczema
M	**M**ucopolysaccharidoses
A I	**A**drenal **I**nsufficiency
D	**D**iabetes insipidus

NB The AID in Maid = HIV

E. False-negative sweat test

Sweet**PEA**s aren't nuts (aren't nots = false negatives)

P	**P**oor technique
E	o**E**dema
A	**A**typical CF

1.4 Miscellaneous

A. Estimating the insertion distance of an endotracheal tube based on a baby's weight

1, 2, 3, 4 . . . 7, 8, 9, 10

1 kg	insert to	**7** cm
2 kg	insert to	**8** cm
3 kg	insert to	**9** cm
4 kg	insert to	**10** cm

B. Meconium aspiration syndrome (MAS)

MAS MASHes Lungs

M   **M**acrophages (ie inflammation)
A   **A**irway Obstruction and **A**sphyxia
S   **S**urfactant inactivation
H   **H**ypoxia, **H**ypercarbia, **H⁺** (acidosis), **H**ypertension

NB We can expand the A segment further by thinking in terms of what happens to the **A**ir in an airway:

As a result of obstruction the air can:

Leave and not get back in	**A**telectasis
Escape outside of the airways	**A**ir leak
Get into an airway and not get out	**A**ir trapping

---

notes

MAS affects approximately 5% of neonates born with meconium stained liquor.

Meconium is rarely passed before 37 weeks gestation, hence MAS is generally a condition affecting term or post-term infants.

50% of infants with MAS require ventilation.

The mortality is 5–12%.

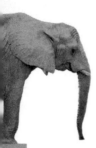

2. Cardiovascular paediatrics

2.1 Causes of cyanosis in congenital cyanotic heart disease

A. 6Ts

Transposition of the great arteries
Tricuspid atresia
Total anomalous pulmonary venous drainage
Truncus arteriosus
Tetralogy of Fallot's
Pulmonary a**T**resia

B. 0, 1, 2, 3, 4, 5

0   0 pulmonaries = pulmonary atresia
1   Only 1 big vessel = truncus arteriosus
2   2 vessels wrong way round = transposition
3   'Tri' = tricuspid atresia
4   tetra = tetralogy
5   Five letters = TAPVD (**T**otal **A**nomalous **P**ulmonary **V**enous **D**rainage)

2.2 ECG changes

A. Bundle branch block

ECG pattern shown in right bundle branch block = **MaRRoW**
ECG pattern shown in left bundle branch block = **WiLLiaM**
MaRRoW   **M** pattern in V1 and **W** in V6 in **R**ight
WiLLiaM   **W** pattern in V1 and M in V6 in **L**eft

B. Hypokalaemia

No POT No Tea

No **pot**assium causes depressed **T** waves

2.3 Miscellaneous mnemonics

A. Causes of hypertension

CREEPS make my BP soar

C	**C**oarctation
R	**R**enal
E	**E**ndocrine
E	**E**ssential
P	**P**haeochromocytoma

> **notes**
>
> Hypertension is defined as an elevation of blood pressure above the 95th centile.
>
> Occurs in 1–3% of children.
>
> Essential hypertension is rare in children whereas it accounts for most cases of hypertension in adults.
>
> Endocrine causes include: **C**onn's syndrome, **C**ushings syndrome, **C**AH and phaeo**C**hromo**C**ytoma. = All C's.

B. Acute rheumatic fever

I spilt Noodles in SYD and ARTHur's MERRY MULTICOLOURED CAR

(I spilt)

Noodles	**N**odules
SYD	**SYD**enham's chorea
ARTH	**ARTH**ritis
Merry multicoloured	Erythema multiforme
Car	**CAR**ditis

> **notes**
>
> Inflammatory condition occurring in response to group A beta haemolytic streptococcal infection.
>
> Initial infection is followed by the above manifestations up to 2–6 weeks later.
>
> Diagnosis is made on the basis of the Duckett Jones criteria.
>
> Two major features or one major and two minor features are required along with evidence of a recent streptococcal infection.
>
> Major features: Carditis, polyarthritis, Sydenham's chorea, erythema marginatum, subcutaneous nodules.
>
> Minor features: fever, arthralgia, Long PR interval on ECG, Raised ESR/CRP, leucocytosis.

C. Causes of pulmonary stenosis
WARNED

Williams
Alagilles
Rubella
Noonan's
Ehlers–**D**anlos

D. Holt Oram syndrome

Think of the condition as **HOLE't Oram**

It is associated with **holes**, ie ASDs and VSDs

E. Marfan's syndrome

Think of the first three letters **MAR**

Mitral and **a**ortic **r**egurgitation

F. Congenital Rubella

Gentle Mr. Ella bought a 3-piece suite

Gentle (Mr.) Ella	**Congenital** Rubella and **M**itral **R**egurgitation
3-Piece suite	**3 Ps** Patent ductus arteriosus (**PDA**) and **P**eripheral **P**ulmonary stenosis

G. Diagnosis of Kawasaki's disease

My HEART

M   **M**ucosal
H   **H**and extremity change
E   **E**ye changes
A   **A**denopathy
R   **R**ash
T   **T**emperature

NB This mnemonic also helps you remember that the heart is also affected

H. Side-effects of prostaglandin (PGE_1)

The five Fs

Forget to breath
Fever
Flushing
Fits
Flutter, ie tachycardia

I. VSD v ASD Which is commoner?

VSD is **V**ery common

ASD is **A**lmost as common

J. Types of VSD

Mnemonic: **PODIUM**

Perimembranous
Outlet
Doubly committed
Inlet
Unaligned (actually malaligned)
Muscular

K. Causes of methaemoglobinaemia

Mnemonic: **CANN** I meet a haemogoblin?

Congenital
Aniline dyes
Nitrites
Nitrobenzene

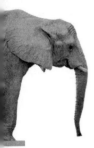

3. Paediatric neurology

3.1 Basic anatomy

A. Reflexes

1, 2, 3, 4, 5, 6, 7, 8

Ankle S**1**, S**2**
Knee L**3**, L**4**
Biceps C**5**, C**6**
Triceps C**7**, C**8**

A more memorable type 3 mnemonic goes as follows:

S1, 2   Buckle my shoe
L3, 4   Kick on my door
C5, 6   Pick up sticks
C7, 8   Put the latch on the gate

B. Innervation of the diaphragm

3, 4, 5 keeps your diaphragm alive

The innervation of the diaphragm is by C3, 4, 5

3.2 Symptoms, signs and causes

A. Causes of a coma

AEIOU

A	**A**poplexy	A slightly more refined word for stroke
E	**E**pilepsy	
I	**I**nfection	
O	**O**xygen (not a cause itself but severe asphyxia can be)	
U	**U**raemia (representing all metabolic causes)	

> **notes**
>
> NB Avoid having too many mnemonics beginning with AEIOU as this will lead to confusion.
>
> The causes of a coma are legion, but it helps to have a ready-to-made list at your hand of the broad-brush causes.

B. Scanning speech abnormality

DANISH women make me tremble

D	**D**ysdiadochokinesis
A	**A**taxia
N	**N**ystagmus
I	**I**ntention tremor
S	**S**peech
H	**H**ypotonia

C. Signs of white matter disorders (eg Krabbe's, metachromatic leukodystrophy etc)

SOAP (which is also white!)

S	**S**pasticity/**S**eizures
O	**O**ptic atrophy
A	**A**taxia
P	**P**eripheral neuropathy

D. Causes of a cherry red spot

The Farmer Picks the GM cherries out of his Sack

Farmer	**F**arber's
Picks	Niemann–**Pick**
GM	**GM** 1
Sack	Tay **Sach**'s

> **notes**
>
> All the above are lysosomal enzyme disorders.
>
> Cherry red spots appear when retinal ganglion cells in the parafoveal region accumulate excess material causing them to swell and burst. The red spot is essentially the revealed colour of the normal fundus.
>
> Reference: Fenichel, G.M. *Clinical Pediatric Neurology. A Signs and Symptoms Approach*. Elsevier Saunders. 5th edition.

E. Assessment of neurological state

AVPU

- **A** **A**lert
- **V** Responds to **V**oice
- **P** Responds to **P**ain
- **U** **U**nresponsive

> **note**
>
> NB This is a simpler and quicker assessment to do than the Glasgow coma score.

3.3 Miscellaneous

A. Prophylaxis of migraine

P for prophylaxis; **P** for the drugs

- **P** **P**ropanolol
- **P** **P**izotifen

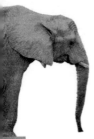

4. Fluids/renal

4.1 Basic knowledge

A. Fluid regimens

4, 2, 1

For children over 10 kg:
For the first 10 kg they need **4** ml·kg⁻¹·h⁻¹
For the next 10 kg they need **2** ml·kg⁻¹·h⁻¹
Thereafter per kg they need **1** ml·kg⁻¹·h⁻¹

For example a 22 kg child requires:

4mls/hr for each kg of the first 10 kg 40mls/hr
2mls/hr for each kg of the next 10kg 20mls/hr
1ml/hr for each kg thereafter 2mls/hr

total requirement 62mls/hr

B. Causes of hypokalaemia

A, B, C, D, E, F, G

A	**A**lkalosis
B	**B**₂ agonists/**B**artter's syndrome
C	**C**ushing's/**C**onn's
D	**D**iuretics/diuresis/distal RTA drugs
E	**E**xtrarenal losses (ie intestinal)
F	**F**anconi syndrome
G	**G**itelman's syndrome

NB Proximal and distal RTAs can both cause hypokalaemia.

C. Causes of hyperkalaemia

FRAMES

F   **F**ailure (renal)
R   **R**habdomyolysis
A   **A**ddison's
M   **M**etabolic acidosis
E   **E**xcess administration
S   **S**pironolactone

D. Features of hypercalcaemia

Stones, bones, groans, psychic moans

Stones	Renal stones
Bones	Lytic lesions
Groans	Abdominal pain
Psychic moans	Depression

E. Causes of hypercalcaemia.

Mnemonic: **H**igh **5** Is

Hyperparathyroidism
Idiopathic
Infantile
Infections
Infiltrations
Ingestion
Skeletal disorders

Infections: Tuberculosis

Infiltrations: malignancy, sarcoidosis

Ingestions: Milk-alkali syndrome, thiazide diuretics, Vitamin intoxication

Skeletal disorders: Hypophosphatasia, immobilisation, skeletal dysplasias

F. Cystinuria; amino acids not reabsorbed by the proximal tubule

COAL

C   **C**ystine
O   **O**rnithine
A   **A**rginine
L   **L**ysine

> **notes**
>
> Incidence 1:650
>
> Inborn error leading to failure to resorb some amino acids leading to increased Excretion in the urine.
>
> Clinically <3% of patients are affected with renal calculi.

G. Causes of haematuria

He's Pee'd V PINTS of blood

V (5)   **V**ascular
P   **P**arenchymal
I   **I**nfection
N   **N**eoplasia
T   **T**rauma
S   **S**tones/**s**ystemic

> **notes**
>
> Haematuria is a relatively common presenting symptom/sign of renal disease.
>
> Haematuria can be classified as macroscopic and microscopic.
>
> There is a 0.5–1.6% prevalence of asymptomatic microscopic haematuria in school children.
>
> Urinary tract infection is the commonest cause.

H. Causes of a low C3/C4

Snaps and slaps get reduced complements

SNaps   **Sh**unt **N**ephritis
SLaps   **S**ystemic **L**upus erythematosus
sl**APS**   **A**cute **P**ost **S**treptococcal glomerulonephritis

I. Causes of a metabolic acidosis with a high anion gap

Mnemonic: **I see (C) MUDPILES**

I   Isoniazid
C   Cyanide
M   Methanol, metformin
U   Uraemia
D   Diabetic ketoacidosis
P   Paraldehyde
I   Iron, Inborn error of metabolism
L   Lactic acidosis
E   Ethanol, ethylene glycol
S   Salicylates

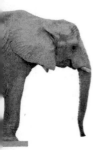

5. Immunology

5.1 The immunoglobulins

A. Immunoglobulin types
GAMED

Each letter stands for a type

B. Which immunoglobulin crosses the placenta?
G gravitates across during Gestation

5.2 Conditions

A. Wiskott Aldrich Syndrome
11 Ex-PET WASPs bit me!

11x	The gene is located on chromosome X position **11**
P	**P**latelets (low)
E	**E**czema
T	**T** cell abnormalities
WASPS	Abnormal gene is **W**iskott **A**ldrich **S**yndrome **P**rotein

> **notes**
>
> Wiskott Aldrich syndrome.
>
> X linked recessive.
>
> Gene defect in the WASP protein at position Xp11.
>
> As well as thrombocytopaenia and eczema patients are at risk of severe life threatening infections autoimmune problems and malignancies (lymphoma.).

B. Treatment of severe T cell disorders

T   **T** for   transplant (bone marrow)

C. Di George Syndrome

CATCH 22

C   **C**ardiac abnormalities
A   **A**bnormal facies
T   **T**hymic abnormality   **T** cell abnormalities
C   **C**left palate
H   **H**ypocalcaemia
22 Microdeletions are on chromosome **22**
        (position 11 – remember, its half of 22)

D. Types of hypersensitivity reactions

Mnemonic: **ACID**

Anaphylactic (I)
Cytotoxic-mediated (II)
Immune complex (III)
Delayed hypersensitivity (IV)

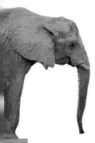

6. Gastrointestinal

6.1 Causes of obstruction

'Inside, outside, wall'

This is a way of categorising and thinking about different causes of obstruction. It is usually used for obstructions in the GI tract but can actually be expanded for use when considering obstructions anywhere else.

Essentially any symptom due to a GI blockage can be the result of obstruction within the lumen of the bowel (ie 'inside'), intramurally (ie within the bowel wall) or extrinsic compression of the bowel (ie 'outside').

For example, constipation can be due to:

Inside   Compacted faecal matter; stricture
Outside   Intra-abdominal tumour, eg neuroblastoma, adhesions
Wall   Intestinal tumour (rare).

This can easily be amended for use outside the GI tract however. Consider for example the causes of a wheeze which we have met before.

Inside   Foreign body, mucus (infection)
Outside   Vascular rings, enlarged thyroid
Wall   Anaphylaxis (oedema).

6.2 Symptoms signs and causes

A. Abdominal distension
The 5 Fs

F	**F**latus
F	**F**at
F	**F**luid
F	**F**aeces
F	**F**etus

In adults fibroids are added in as a sixth F.

B. Causes of hepatomegaly
CHIMPS are great big Lovers

C	**C**onnective tissue disorders
H	**H**aematological
I	**I**nfective
M	**M**etabolic
P	**P**arenchymal
S	**S**ystemic

Lovers   Livers

These are also the categories for splenomegaly and hepatosplenomegaly.

> **note**
>
> When asked 'Tell me, what are the causes of hepatomegaly?' It always looks more impressive to say 'Well Professor, the causes of hepatomegaly can be divided up into connective tissue disorders, haematological . . . the most commonest of which are . . . ' as this shows evidence of your ability to systematise and order your thinking.

C. Signs of pyloric stenosis

remember the 3 Ps

P   **P**alpable mass
P   **P**eristalsis
P   **P**rojectile vomiting

(Potassium is also low)

> **notes**
>
> Presents between 2–7 weeks of age generally.
>
> Biochemical features include a hypochloraemic, hypokalaemic metabolic acidosis.
>
> The projectile vomiting is non-bile stained.

D. Unusual causes of gastrointestinal bleeding

Don't forget the **3 Hs**

HUS   **H**aemolytic–uraemic syndrome
HDN   **H**aemorrhagic disease of the newborn
HSP   **H**enoch–Schonlein Purpura

E. Clinical signs of chronic liver disease

Don't get hep B at the JAP SEX CLUB

J   **J**aundice
A   **A**naemia
P   **P**almar erythema
S   **S**pider naevi
E   **E**ncephalopathy (late sign)
X   **X**anthelasma

CLUB   **CLUB**bing

F. Features of Wilson's disease

C3H3W13

C3 **C**erebellar signs
Corneal **C**ayser Fleischer rings (begins with a K really!)
Copper/**c**eruloplasmin (urinary copper high, serum caeruloplasmin low)

H3 **H**epatosplenomegaly
Haemolytic anaemia
Handwriting deteriorates

W13 Gene is on chromosome **13**

---

notes

Autosomal recessive disease, with the gene localised to chromosome 13.

Incidence 1: 200,000

Caused by reduced synthesis of caerulopasmin and defective excretion of copper in the bile causing accumulation of copper in the liver, brain, kidney and corneas.

Hepatic manifestations include, hepatitis, fulminant disease and portal hypertension.

Renal disease includes renal tubular dysfunction and rickets.

Neurological abnormalities are commoner with increasing age and include worsening school performance, personality change inco-ordination tremor and dysarthria.

Treatment is with penicillamine and zinc to reduce copper absorbtion.

6.3 Miscellaneous

A. Meckel's diverticulum

The rule of 2s

Occurs in **2**% of the population
Male:female ratio is **2**:1
2 inches long
2 feet from the ileocaecal valve in adults

B. Breast milk versus cow's milk

Composition

Women's milk has more **W**hey
Cow's milk has more **C**asein

C. Contraindicated drugs in breastfeeding

BREAST

B   **B**romocriptine
R   **R**adioactive isotopes
E   **E**rgotamine
A   **A**miodarone
S   **S**ex hormones
T   **T**etracyclines

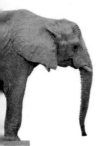

7. Genetics

7.1 How to match conditions to chromosomes

Which chromosome does the gene for cystic fibrosis occur on?

Okay so you know its chromosome 7. But then how about the next question?

Which chromosome does the gene for SMA occur on?

Stumped?

One of the difficulties of the MRCPCH exam is that you are often expected to remember on which chromosome a certain gene for a condition is located. Having to memorise a long list of conditions is a bit of a pain and unfortunately you cannot resort to a deep-learning approach – you just have to memorise these facts.

What follows is a tried and tested method that I have adapted to this onerous chore, and it is known as the loci approach.

To begin, imagine a place that is very well known to you. It might be totally imaginary or it might be the house you grew up in. Picture it very clearly in your mind's eye, and divide the entire place up into 23 separate areas. It helps if you are thinking of a pretty large place that is easily divisible.

Now why have we chosen the number 23?

Well each area/room will represent one chromosome (pair).

At the risk of repeating myself, remember that the areas must be clearly separate from another as you see it. The next step is to take a journey in your mind's eye through each of those rooms, one after the other. When you imagine doing this there must be a clear journey that takes you from the first room representing chromosome 1 to the last room representing chromosome 23.

Now what you are going to do is imagine characters representing various conditions and place them in the appropriate room depending on which chromosome they can be found on.

For example:

William's syndrome.

I was always a *Carry On* fan as a child and I imagine Kenneth Williams with his well known semi-gurning expression standing with the words 'Maaaatronnn' on his lips. The image must be as vivid/rude as possible. Now place Kenneth Williams in room number 7 in your imaginary house, because as you know the gene for William's syndrome is found on chromosome 7.

For each and every condition whose position you want to know, do something similar. The only thing limiting you is your imagination.

After a bit you will realise that some rooms are more crowded than others. The seventh room on your journey for instance, which has not only Kenneth Williams but also a character representing cystic fibrosis. This explains why the rooms must be large enough for your images not to end up blurred and confused.

It will take a bit of practice to get going, but it really does work. Although an initial outlay in terms of time for setting up a 'home' and peopling it with characters is called for, once done you will probably find that you can rapidly and reliably recall which chromosome is associated with a certain abnormality. The important thing is to place characters in the room, go on the journey in a methodical manner, and to do it over and over again until the image is safely fastened onto the relevant room.

7.2 Specific conditions

A. DiGeorge syndrome

CATCH-22

C	**C**ardiac abnormalities
A	**A**bnormal facies
T	**T**hymic absence/abnormality/**T** cell abnormality
C	**C**left palate
H	**H**ypocalcaemia
22	The condition is located on chromosome **22**

> **notes**
>
> Caused by a microdeletion on chromosome 22q.
>
> Features due to developmental defect of the fourth branchial arch.

B. Hurler's syndrome

HURLER's

H	**H**epatosplenomegaly
U	**U**nusual facial features
R	**R**ecessive
L	**L**-iduronidase deficiency
E	**E**yes clouded
R	**R**etardation
S	**S**hort stubby fingers

> **notes**
>
> A mucopolysaccharidosis. One of the lysosomal disorders.
>
> Characterised by defective degradation and storage of mucopolysaccharides (glycosaminoglycans.)

C. Hurler's versus Hunters – which have corneal clouding?

Remember that hunters needs good eyesight so don't have clouding, but hurlers can still hurl objects with corneal clouding!!

D. Marfan's syndrome

MARFAN's

M **M**itral valve prolapse
A **A**ortic aneurysm
R **R**etinal detachment
F **F**ibrillin gene abnormality
A **A**rachnodactyly
N **PN**eumothoraces (spontaneous or apical blebs on CXR)
S **S**keletal abnormality

---

notes

Multisystem disorder caused by a defect in the fibrillin gene on chromosome 15.

Cardiovascular involvement main cause of death.

Diagnosis is based on the Ghent diagnostic criterion, and requires the presence of a family history and major/minor criteria in different organ systems.

E. A common sign in ataxia telangiectasia

AT stands for the first letters of the condition

AT **A**bsent **T**hymus

F. Russell Silver

ABCDEFH

A **A**symmetry
B **B**ossing (frontal)
C **C**linodactyly
D **D**warfism
E **E**xcretion (GU abnormalities)
F **F**acies (triangular)
H **H**ead is large proportionately

A sporadic condition associated with the above features. Asymmetry is the key feature.

They tend to be very fussy eaters and hyperhydrosis has been noted.

Reference: *Oxford Desk reference Clinical Genetics.* Firth, H.V, Hurst J.A. Oxford. First edition.

G. Features of Tay Sach's

SACHS

S **S**pots in the macula
A **A**shkenazi Jews
C **C**NS degeneration
H **H**exosaminidase deficiency
S **S**torage disease

H. Features of Prader-Willi

Mnemonic: 'H3O'

Hyperphagia
Hypotonia
Hypopigmentation
Obesity

Commonest recognised genetic cause of obesity.

Affects 1/10,000 – 1/15,000 children.

Initially infants have hypotonia with poor feeding and failure to thrive.

Rapid weight gain and hyperphagia 2–4 yrs.

An example of genomic imprinting and uniparental disomy.

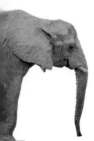

8. Resuscitation and life support

8.1 Miscellaneous

A. Initial basic life support

Prior to initial evaluation adopt a **SAFE** approach

S	**S**hout for help
A	**A**pproach with care
F	**F**ree from danger
E	**E**valuate ABC . . .

B. When undertaking any form of resuscitation remember:

A, B, C, D, E

A	**A**irway
B	**B**reathing
C	**C**irculation
D	**D**isability
E	**E**nvironment

Some say A, B, C . . . **D, E, F, G**

Where **D, E, F, G** is **D**on't **E**ver **F**orget **G**lucose

C. When assessing someone's neurological state remember

AVPU

A	**A**lert
V	**V**oice response
P	**P**ain response
U	**U**nresponsive

D. Causes of pulseless electrical activity

4 (HT)

H	**H**ypoxia
H	**H**ypovolaemia
H	**H**yper/hypokalaemia
H	**H**ypothermia
T	**T**ension pneumothorax
T	**T**amponade
T	**T**oxicity
T	**T**hromboembolism

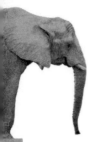

9. Neonatology

9.1 Miscellaneous

A. Circumcision

The five Ms of circumcision

M **M**oses
M **M**ohammad (ie members of the Jewish and Muslim communities)
M **M**aternal reasons
M **M**oney (cynical!)
M **M**edical reasons (controversial!)

B. Estimating the size of the ET tube in neonates

1, 2, 3, 4 . . . 7, 8, 9, 10

Weight (kg)	Length of ETT (cm)
1	7
2	8
3	9
4	10

C. VACTERL syndrome

VACTERL

V **V**ertebral anomalies
A **A**nal
C **C**ardiac
T **T**racheal
E o**E**sophageal
R **R**enal
L **L**imb

> **notes**
>
> Sporadic condition.
>
> Recurrence risk 2–3%
>
> Diagnosis requires one anomaly in each of the three anatomical domains (limb, thorax, pelvis/lower abdomen), or two anomalies in two domains for a probable diagnosis.

D. ABO incompatibility

Which is worse?

O-A or O-B?

B is **B**ad

but

A is **A**wful

E. Causes of persistent pulmonary hypertension of the newborn (PPHN)

DIAPHRAGMATIC

D **D**iaphragmatic hernia **D**rugs
I **I**nfection
A **A**spiration
P **P**ostmaturity
H **H**yperviscosity
R **R**DS
A **A**sphyxia
G **G**rowth retardation
M **M**aternal NSAIDS
A **A**ir leak
T **T**TN
I **I**diopathic
C **C**ongenital anomalies

F. Management of PPHN

SOAPSTONE

S **S**edation and less **s**timulation
O **O**xygen
A **A**cidosis correction
P **P**ressors and volume
S **S**urfactant
T **T**olazoline, Touchless (ie less stimulation)
O **O**scillation
N **N**itric oxide
E **E**CMO

---

notes

PPHN

Also known as persistent fetal circulation.

Is present when an infant with structurally normal heart has:

Severe hypoxaemia, usually a PaO2 <5–6kPa in an FiO2 of 1.0.

Hypoxaemia disproportional to the radiological and clinical abnormality seen. There is often only mild lung disease itself.

Evidence of a right to left shunt.

G. Abnormal nappy colour

i. Blue diaper syndrome

If you're a blue baby you like tripping

This condition is caused by excretion of tryptophan metabolites in the stool.

ii. Pink staining in the nappy

If you're a pink baby, it must be something you ate.

This is caused by urate (you ate) crystals in the urine.

H. Causes of neonatal hepatitis

TORCH

T	**TORCH T**oxoplasmosis
O	**O**ther
R	**R**ubella
C	**C**MV
H	**H**erpes

I. Which is more superficial and mobile, caput succedaneum or cephalhaematoma?

Caput: It's like a cap, therefore superficial and mobile

J. APGAR score

APGAR

A	**A**ppearance
P	**P**ulse
G	**G**rimace
A	**A**ctivity
R	**R**espiratory rate

The traditional way of assessing newborns after delivery.

Devised by Dr. Virginia Apgar in 1953.

Each feature is graded with a score of 0,1 or 2.

Scored traditionally at 1, 5 and 10 minutes of age (and longer if needed).

K. Features associated with drug withdrawal in the neonate

Mnemonic: '**Withdrawal**'

W Wakefulness
I Irritability
T Tremulousness
H Hyperactivity
D Diarrhoea
R Rub marks
A Apnoea's
W Weight loss
A Alkalosis
L Lacrimation

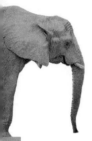

10. Sepsis

10.1 General mnemonics

A. The commonest cause of septic arthritis

SA stands for septic arthritis and *Staphylococcus aureus*

B. Croup

5 Ss

- **S** Subglottic swelling
- **S** Stridor
- **S** Seal-like cough
- **S** Steroids first-line treatment
- **S** Sympathomimetics; in particular adrenaline

C. Drugs used to treat Tuberculosis

Mnemonic **RIPES**

- **R** Rifampicin
- **I** Isoniazid
- **P** Pyrazinadmide
- **E** Ethambutol
- **S** streptomycin

D. Measles

4 Cs

Cough
Coryza
Conjunctivitis
Koplik Spots (sounds like a 'c')

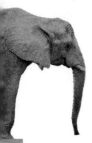

11. Statistics

11.1 Statistics

A. Sensitivity and specificity

SNnOUT and SPpIN

If a test for a condition with high sensitivity (**SN**) is negative (**n**), it rules **OUT** the condition. If a test for a condition with high specificity (**SP**) is positive (**p**) it rules **IN** the condition.

B. Distinguishing type I and type II errors

A type I error is essentially a false-positive result (ie a trial which finds a difference between a drug and placebo when in fact there is no difference at all).

Remember it is a false result first of all by virtue of the fact that it is an error.

Remember it is a false-positive result because:

Type I . . . draw a little curl on the **I** gives us a **P** (positive).

A type II error is essentially a false-negative result (ie a trial which finds no difference between a drug and placebo when in fact there was a difference).

Again, remember it is false by virtue of the fact that it is an error.

Remember it is a false-negative result because

Type II . . . if we add a bar diagonally to the **II** it becomes an **N** (negative).

The probability of committing a type II error is called the **BETA** value. Beta is the second letter of the Greek alphabet, hence represents a type II error!

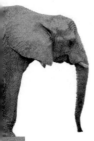

12. Rheumatology

12.1 Miscellaneous

A. Features of systemic onset juvenile chronic arthritis

FRESH SALMON

F Fever
R Rash (**salmon** pink)
E ESR high
S Serositis
H Hepatitis/hepatomegaly

S Splenomegaly
A Arthritis
L Lymphadenopathy
M Malaise
O Ouch (pain)
N Normochromic normocytic anaemia.

(**N**egative for rheumatoid factor)

(**N**egative for anti-nuclear antibodies)

> **notes**
>
> Juvenile chronic arthritis.
>
> Commonest chronic rheumatic illness in children.
>
> Diagnosis made in children under 16, with arthritis for at least 6 weeks without any other identifiable cause.
>
> Systemic form accounts for 10–20% of the total.

B. Conditions associated with being HLA-B27 positive

By 27 you're a-losing the right to react to cute cyclists, beware even old crones will leave you sore

a-losing	An**kylosing** spondylitis
right	**Reiter's** syndrome
react	**react**ive arthritis
cute cyclists	acute iridocyclitis
crones	inflammatory bowel disease (Crohn's)
sore	psoriasis

C. Commonest cause of septic arthritis

Remember the first letters of the condition.

SA *S*taphylococcus *a*ureus

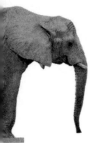

13. Endocrinology

13.1 Miscellaneous

A. Puberty

8, 9, 10, 12, 13, 14

<8 years in girls   Abnormal puberty
<9 years in boys   Abnormal puberty
10 years in girls   Average age of puberty
12 years in boys   Average age of puberty
13 years in girls   Delayed puberty
14 years in boys   Delayed puberty

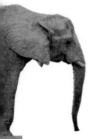

14. Psychiatry

14.1 Autism

A. Characteristic features

SCARE

Social interactions
Communication
Activities restricted and
Repetitive
Early onset

B. Autism and IQ

Approximately:

50% have an IQ below 50
70% have an IQ below 70
100% have an IQ below 100

14.2 Anorexia nervosa and bulimia

A. Anorexia

Features begin with **A** (A for anorexia)

Avoidance of food especially fattening ones
Altered body image
Amenorrhoea
Anxiety/fear of weight gain

B. Bulimia

Bulimia is characterised by among other things **b**inging

14.3 Substance abuse

The **CRAFFT** screen

C **C**ar. Have you driven a car (or taken a ride) under the influence of drugs?

R **R**elax. Do you use drugs or alcohol to relax?

A **A**lone. Do you use drugs or alcohol when you are alone?

F **F**orget. Do you sometimes forget what you did while using drugs/alcohol?

F **F**amily/friends. Do they ever tell you to cut down on your use?

T **T**rouble. Have you got into trouble while using drugs?

> **notes**
>
> This is a six-item screening test for adolescent substance abuse. Two or more yes answers indicates significant abuse with >90% sensitivity and >80% specificity.

14.4 Attention deficit hyperactivity disorder (ADHD)

A. Characteristic features of ADHD

Remember the 'six **I**s'

Inattention
Increased activity
Impulsiveness
Impairment in multiple settings
Inappropriate (for developmental stage)
Incessant

ADHD is a neurodevelopmental/behavioural disorder characterised by inattention, impulsiveness and hyperactivity (increased activity). It is seen in multiple settings, such as at home and at school. The behaviour is inappropriate for the child's developmental age and persistent for more than 6 months.

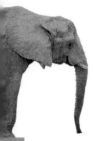

15. Dermatology

15.1 Causes of acute urticaria

The five Is

Infection
Infestation
Ingestion
Injections
Inhalation

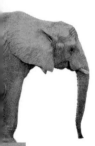

16. Emergency medicine

16. Ingested substances that are opaque on X-ray

CHIPS

Chloral hydrate
Heavy metals
Iodides
Phenothiazines, **P**sychotropics
Slow release capsules

16.2 Features of organophosphate poisoning

SLUDGE and DUMBELS

Salivation
Lacrimation
Urination
Defecation
Gastrointestinal cramps
Emesis

Defecation
Urination
Miosis
Bradycardia
Emesis
Lacrimation
Salivation

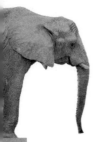

17. Pharmacology

17.1 Side-effects of corticosteroids

CUSHINGOID MAP

Cataracts
Ulcers
Striae
Hypertension
Infection risk
Necrosis (avascular) of bone
Growth retardation
Osteoporosis
Increased intracranial pressure
Diabetes mellitus

Myopathy
Adipose tissue hypertrophy
Pancreatitis

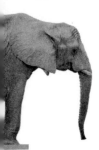

18. Paediatric surgery

18.1 Umbilical herniae in children

The rule of 3s

3% of live births
3:1000 need repair
Repair done after age of **3**

18.2 Meckel's diverticulum

The rule of 2s

Occurs in **2%** of the population
2:1 male: female ratio
2 inches long and **2** feet from ileocaecal junction in ADULTS
1:**2** contain ectopic tissue
2% are symptomatic

18.3 Complications of undescended testes

TESTIS

Trauma
Epididymo-orchitis
Sterility
Torsion
Intestinal hernia
Seminoma

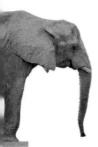

19. Orthopaedics

19.1 When to be concerned

Children who present with the 5 Ss

Symptoms
Stiffness
A**S**ymmetry
Syndromes
Systemic disorders

19.2 The limping child

DIPS

Age (years)	Condition
Birth	**D**evelopmental dysplasia
	Infection
5–9	**P**erthes disease
10–15	**S**lipped upper femoral epiphyses

19.3 Risk factors for congenital dislocation of the hip

6 Fs

First born
Female
Funny presentation (breech)
Family history
Fluid deficiency (oligohydramnios)
Fat (large child)

19.4 Features of osteopetrosis

MARBLES

Multiple fractures
Anaemia
Restricted cranial nerves
Blindness and deafness
Liver enlarged
Erlenmeyer flask deformity
Splenomegaly

19.5 Incidences of paediatric orthopaedic conditions

1/1000, 1/10,000, 1/100,000

1/1000 Congenital dislocation of the hip (CDH), metatarsus adductus

1/10,000 Perthes disease

1/100,000 Slipped femoral epiphyses

19.6 The patient with a suspected fracture

Assess the 5 Ps

Pain
Pulse
Pallor
Paraesthesia
Paralysis

> **note**
>
> These are vital features to look for as they signal impending or established compartment syndrome.

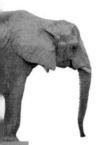

20. Haematology/ Oncology

20.1 Causes of aplastic anaemia

(IP) 3

Infection
Immune disease
Irradiation
Pregnancy
Paroxysmal nocturnal haemoglobinuria
Preleukaemia

20.2 Causes of an anterior mediastinal mass seen on imaging studies

Five Ts

Teratoma
Thymoma
Thyroid tumour
T cell leukaemia
Terrible lymphoma

20.3 Diencephalic syndrome

The 3 Es

Euphoria
Emaciation
Emesis

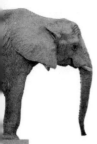

21. Miscellaneous

21.1 Taking a pain history

SOCRATES

Site
Onset
Character
Radiation/relieving factors
Associated factors
Treatment
Exacerbating factors
Severity

21.2 Reading an X-ray

ABCs

Appropriateness/**A**dequacy/**A**lignment
Bones
Cartilage
Soft tissues

21.3 General differential diagnosis

TIN CAN BED

Trauma
Infection/**I**nflammation/**I**diopathic/**I**atrogenic
Neoplastic

Congenital
Arteriovenous
Nutritional

Biochemical
Endocrine
Degenerative/drug induced

Mnemonic index

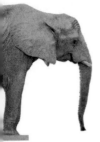

Subject index

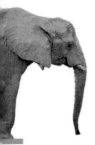

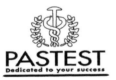